THE

POCKET DIETITIAN

(1918)

Or, How to Combine Food for Correct Eating. Self-Help for the Sick and Those with Cranky Stomachs. Special Menus for Summer and Winter.

J.H. Tilden

ISBN 1-56459-871-3

Kessinger Publishing's Rare Reprints
Thousands of Scarce and Hard-to-Find Books!

- •
- •
- •
- •
- •
- •
- •
- •
- •
- •
- •
- •
- •
- •
- •
- •
- •
- •
- •

We kindly invite you to view our extensive catalog list at:
http://www.kessinger.net

Warning—Disclaimer

It is exceedingly difficult to secure an honest hearing or any criticism of authority. Established beliefs are well nigh invulnerable because they are accorded infallibility by the masses who are educated to believe that they will be damned for thinking, and because of this, few will tolerate opposition of any nature to anything they have been educated to believe. People who have their thinking done for them are always intolerant."

—*J. H. Tilden, M.D.*

Acknowledgment

My indebtedness to Miss Frieda B. Gantz for arranging the matter for this booklet is hereby acknowledged.

It is one thing to dictate material for a book, and quite another thing to make a book out of the material. Order is the first law of nature, and books without order have no power to grip the student.

Preface

Dr. John H. Tilden, the son of a physician, was born in Van Burenburg, Illinois, on January 21, 1851. He received his medical education at the Eclectic Medical Institute, Cincinnati, Ohio, a medical school founded in 1830 as a protest against the allopathic and homeopathic schools of medicine of that time. He was graduated in 1872, with the degree of doctor of medicine. From the best information we can obtain, his father was a Dr. Joseph G. Tilden, who came from Vermont in 1837 to Kentucky, in which State he married.

Dr. John H. Tilden started the practice of medicine at Nokomis, Illinois, then for a year at St. Louis, Missouri, and then at Litchfield, Illinois, until 1890, when he moved to Denver, Colorado. In Denver he located in the downtown business section, in an office with other doctors. Later he established a sanitarium in an outer section of the city. This sanitarium and school he conducted until 1924, when he sold the Institution, for about half of what he had plowed back into its development, to a Dr. Arthur Voss of Cincinnati, Ohio, intending to devote himself to writing and lecturing. However, he soon became discontented without his school and after a period he bought two residences on Pennsylvania Avenue, in Denver, united them into one and opened a new sanitarium and school, having to borrow from a friend a part of the money with which to make the purchases. This probably was in 1926. This school continued until the Doctor's death, on September 1, 1940.

It was during the early years of his practice in Illinois, that Dr. Tilden began to question the use of medicine to cure illness. His extensive reading, especially of medical studies from European medical schools, and his own thinking, led him to the conclusion that there should be some way to live so as not to build disease, and in this period his thoughts on toxemia began to formulate and materially develop. From the beginning of his practice in Denver, the Doctor used no medicine but practiced his theory of clearing the body of toxic poison and then allowing nature to make the cure, teaching his patients how to live so as not to create a toxic condition and to retain a healthy body free of disease. An uncompromising realist and a strict disciplinarian, the Doctor wasted no time on those who would not relinquish degenerating habits, but to his patients and disciples he was both friend and mentor.

In 1900 he began the publication of a monthly magazine called "The Stuffed Club," which continued until 1915, when he changed the name to "The Philosophy of Health," and in 1926 the name was changed to "Health Review and Critique." His writing for his publication was almost entirely done in the early morning hours, from three until seven. The purpose of the publication was not to make money but to spread knowledge of the Doctor's teachings. In time it attained a wide circulation, not only in this country but also abroad, even in Australia, but it never produced revenue, for the Doctor refused to make it an advertising medium, as often urged to do by advertising firms. As his death revealed, after sixty-eight years of practice, the Doctor had accumulated only an exceedingly modest estate. His life was pre-eminently one of self-sacrifice and of devotion to service, searching after truth, with an indomitable will and with an intense fortitude to adhere to the truth when discovered. In his day the Doctor's thoughts received no support from the established medical profession but brought the strongest of opposition and condemnation.

Frederic N. Gilbert

Foreword

THE Menus which are given in this book are synthetically arranged after the manner of prescribing by Dr. J. H. Tilden, being the quintessence of his many years of practical experience as a dietetic physician. They are wholly adequate for the needs of the people, and more than conform to the recommendations of the Federal Food Administrator. Indeed, it would be most economical, as well as health—and nation-building, if they were followed all the time, in peace no less than in war.

If people would do their "bit" at all times, in conserving food, health, and efficiency, there would be little disease and no wars; there would be no excessive w e a l t h and no squalor; selfishness would give way to honesty and generosity; and charity in the

[5]

form of alms-giving, poor-hospitals and poor-farms, with their poorer service, would soon become extinct. We have no right to impoverish by taking away man's self-respect through donations, gifts, etc. Those who cannot help themselves should be helped to help themselves. Man must be made to stand—not crawl.

Table of Contents

Table of Contents—Continued

The Pocket Dietitian

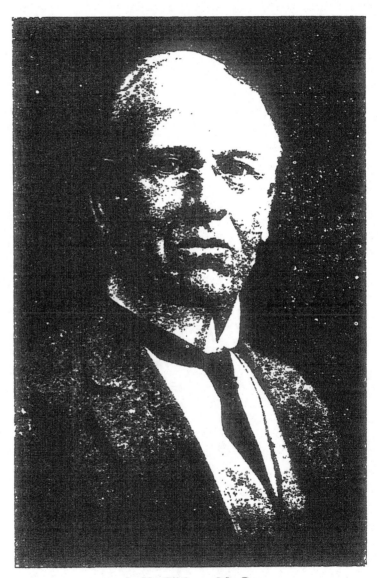

J. H. Tilden, M. D.

INTRODUCTION

Why Diet Cannot Cure

IT IS necessary to disabuse the public mind of a prevailing fallacy regarding the idea that cures can be made by some peculiar diet.

The superstition is universal that disease is an entity, and that entity can be met and vanquished by a fetich —an object, a remedy, something possessed of magical or occult power, such as is ascribed to drugs, vaccines, viruses, and serums.

The modern cures and immunizing agents used by modern medical science are as absurd as the cures and charms of the doctors and witches of one or two hundred years ago. The fundamental principles are the same; only, we of today are not so crude in our manipulations, our technique, and our conceits.

Disease today is believed to be as much of a thing-in-itself—an entity— as at any time in the history of man. And the learned doctors are chasing after the elixir of life—mysterious remedies—as vehemently as ever before, and are as absurdly dogmatic with their newly discovered cures—ephemeral remedies which scarce last over night—as at any time in the history of the world. As proof that these statements are true, I refer to the iteration and reiteration of the medical faculties of the great advance made in the cure of disease—the wonder of bacteriology and surgery. The former, up to date, has not one proven leg on which to stand, and the latter has a vandalized—a mutilated—race of people to show for its merits. The race suicide that has been taking place in the past forty years was inaugurated by surgical specialism. Dr. Battey former of Rome, Georgia, and later of New York City, set the profession agog over normal ovariotomy—oophorectomy; and since the acme of Battey's fame was reached, women have been mutilated by the thousands every year. The fad was assisted mightily by woman herself. When she learned that she could, without danger to life, have the responsibility of motherhood forever removed, she joined the surgeon (who was willing to unsex her because the great Battey, backed by the consensus of surgical opinion, had discovered that *the ovaries were the cause of nearly all the aches and pains of womanhood*) in his war on the disease-producing organ.

After the collapse of Battey's cure-all for women came Tait and hysterectomy (removal of the womb or all the reproductive organs), which was another cure-all for women—particularly those suffering with fibroid tumors. Then came appendicectomy (removal of the appendix); and removal of one after another of all the other organs of the body followed in rapid procession. All of these operations have been, and most of them are now, worked overtime; and all together amount to wholesale vandalism, which is proved unnecessary by the rapid changing of the surgical fashions, with repudiations, recantations, etc.

Unfortunate indeed was the discovery that surgical operations could be successfully performed if they were made aseptically. At first antiseptics were used in surgery in the belief that the drug would kill the germ and render the wound aseptic (free from germs). But it later developed that the real cause of aseptic operations was cleanliness. Before this idea took hold of the professional mind the mortality was made great in surgery from drug poisoning.

The misfortune in discovering aseptic surgery is that it encourages unscrupulous professional men to make unnecessary operations. This forces surgeons who would be conservative into operating, on the questionable principle that "If I do not operate, someone less qualified will." As a result the practice of modern surgery amounts to wholesale vandalism, and the mortality from it far exceeds—yes multiplies many times—the number of deaths that would take place were there not a surgeon on earth. The argument is put forth that fine surgery is needed—that the people could not dispense with skilled surgery— and modern skill justifies the abuse. Those who argue from this side of the question must also declare that drugs, like alcohol, morphine, opium, and other narcotics, justify the wholesale inebriety (ruined lives) which they cause, because of the relief they give to suffering humanity. This is a sentimentalism that has no foundation in truth, and is successfully disputed by all drugless healing systems. The truth is that, when the sick are treated rationally, there is no room, excuse, or need for drugs. And there is no exception to the rule—no, not even syphilis makes an exception. The Mosaic history of the Jews refutes the modern teachings regarding syphilis. All history refutes it .

Many people of knowledge and experience, who concede that drugs are not necessary to the successful treatment of disease in general, make an exception of syphilis. In doing so, they annul and make void all their defense of drug·ess healing. If drugs are a benefit and necessary in any sickness, they are necessary in all—there can be no exception to natural law. Nature can eliminate all intoxication. thereby restoring lost energy, if all depressing and intoxicating habits are given up.

Every poison is a toxin or an intoxicant. Toxins are developed by fermentation and decomposition of all kinds of food stuffs taken in excess of digestive power. Alcohol, tobacco, tea, coffee, and drugs for relieving pain are toxic; which means that they are stimulating—intoxicating—and, when habitually used, bring on enervation and pave the way for affections of all

[15]

kinds, especially those to which there is a predisposition through inheritance. Diseases or affections cannot be cured except by giving up the habit, whatever it is, that enervates; after which lost energy will be restored and full health return.

This argument may be extended to every toxic influence to which man subjects himself; and the conclusion must be the same, namely: A palliation—a fleeting stimulation—that vivifies the body and electrifies the mind does so at the expense of the integrity of the nervous system. All such comforts and pleasures use up nerve energy and bring about early disintegration. Then the question is: Does it pay to handicap efficiency and bring about, in many, nerve bankruptcy, just to secure a fleeting, questionable advantage? Tobacco, coffee, tea, and like stimulants belong to the toxin class. Because someone has managed to live to eighty or ninety years of age who used one or more of these stimulants by virtue of the fact that his organs, on which these stimulants spend their force, started life one hundred per cent efficient, is no proof that all people do the same. Indeed, those with an inherited heart weakness will be, and are, driven into early heart and circulatory affections by the use of these stimulants.

Life is not told in years, but in how much one has lived. A great store of knowledge, gleaned from books and laboratory work and the experiments of others, may make a very full life; but if attainments have not been tested by the acid of experience, the great load of knowledge may not be true. Nothing can mark a greater failure than a life of eighty or ninety years loaded down by conventional lies, and not one record of having refuted one in all those years.

A life that has not honestly investigated popular beliefs to find out if they are true or not, but has accepted on the authority of school, creed, or custom, is a failure, even if it has gone to a hundred. No life is a failure that has wrestled with nature, as Jacob wrestled for Israel, and refused to give up until blessed by an analyzing vision of truth itself. A life that has wrested from nature one truth is greater, if closed at thirty, than a life prolonged to ninety that has refused to investigate and search for truth

It is sufficient to be able to say that everyone of any reputation believes as I do. Indeed, a long time ago all men of respectability and education believed the world flat.

To perform successfully an unnecessary operation, and then grow a conscience that makes its possessor dec'are that such vandalism is both successful and scientific, certainly smacks of superstition and fetichism equal to the days of witchcraft.

Among the more enlightened there is a growing belief that there is no disease; that what is known as disease is nothing more than impaired health —health being a normal standard of well-being—and any lowering of this standard, from work, worry, or improper living, is called disease.

When the cause of disease is taken out of the realm of mysticism and placed on the solid rock of cause and effect, in keeping with man's daily experience with nature, then truth begins to supplant fallacy; understanding begins to repudiate the idea of disease as an entity, and to establish the great truth that the state of man called health is his normal state and his true inheritance, and that disease is that same state handicapped by ignorance and evil customs.

[18]

The idea that cures can be made, if the right remedy can be found, is so mentally ingrained that a second Savior will be required to teach the world that there is no disease *per se;* that what we call disease is impaired health, brought on from wrong thinking and acting.

The people have been taught that there is disease and that there are remedies. This teaching has resulted in their being educated into thinking in the language of disease and remedies, which is fundamentally a fallacy—a fallacy on which is built an ethics that fills the world with hospitals and eleemosynary institutions, which are peopled to overflowing with patients, the majority of whom are in truth monomaniacs, their mania being a belief in disease, and a belief that cures are peculiar to doctors and hospitals. This idea is so firmly established that, when the use of drugs is given up, other cures or Saviors must take their place. The people are not ready to give up one cure-all until safely possessed of another. They go hunting for cures, and the fetiches which they adopt are in keeping with their state of development. A rag on a bush by a sacred well; a charm in the pocket; a blessed handkerchief worn next to the body over the disease; a peculiar prayer; the sacrifice of different organs of the body to the Moloch of surgery; vaccination, and immunization on that order, are all believed to charm away microscopic enemies of mankind. When these and many other superstitions all fail, and the seekers after some peculiar, mysterious, and hidden cure hear of *diet cures*, they are encouraged to look for the mysterious power in food.

What is Health?
TRUTH IS TOO SIMPLE

The idea that all that is necessary to prevent and cure disease is to live simply, rationally, and sensibly, is too simple to be true. The most enlightened fall down and worship anything that is supposed to be potentized by the mysterious entity called cure. This childish aboriginalism fails to bring the blush of shame even to the cheeks of the leading educators of earth. The fact is that civilization is mentally bucked and gagged and delivered over to superstition.

All that is necessary to have health is to live moderately, avoiding excess in work, eating, and sensual pleasures, which, when indulged in to excess, injure digestion, assimilation, and nutrition. The innate developing processes—vital processes—of the body are quite sufficient to right themselves, when wrong, if permitted to do so, by correcting any errors of life that are lowering the health and life standard. This idea is so unlike our inherited and acquired superstitions on the subject of disease and cure that it is necessary, in launching this little DIETITIAN, to protest at its very beginning that in no sense of the word are its teachings on dieting or eating correctly to be construed medicinally, remedially, or in the sense of a cure. All that eating correctly, and taking proper care of the body, is supposed to do, is to keep those well who are in health, or to allow the body to right itself after it has been forced out of normality by wrong eating and wrong life in general. The body will stay normal if properly cared for; and when sick, nothing cures except nature!

Simply live right, and health will follow as a natural sequence. When uncomfortable, or short on physical or mental efficiency, adopt right living, and the body will soon readjust itself —come back to the normal.

[21]

If life is a failure—if success has failed to reward honest, conscientious labor—there must be something wrong with the manner of living. Probably the wits are wool-gathering from toxin poisoning. It may be that thinking is not logical because of the perverting influence of overstimulation. Possibly the manner of living is enervating. If so, the point of view is wrong.

Seek first health and all else will be added. Do not seek by the medicine route, or through some foolish curing scheme that is to make man well without separating him from his bad habits. Remove the cause, and health will follow. If eating is wrong, certainly none except the sensual will expect a cure while bad habits are practiced.

———◆———

Ninety-nine out of every hundred medical facts are medical lies, and medical doctrines are for the most part stark, staring nonsense.— Prof. Gregory, M. D., Edinburgh.

Chapter I.
Foods

FOOD, AS FOUND ON THE MARKET, CONTAINS

```
                   ┌ Water
┌ Edible portion   │                         ┌ Protein
│  —e. g., flesh   │            ┌ Nutrients ─┤ Carbohydrates
│  of meat, yolk   │                         │ Fats
│  and white of    └                         └ Mineral Salts
│  e g g, flour,
│  etc.
│
│ Refuse — e. g.,
│   b o n e s. en-
│   trails, shells,
└   bran, etc.
```

USES OF NUTRIENTS IN THE BODY

*Protein:** Forms tissues; e. g., white (albumin) of eggs, curd (casein) of milk, lean meat, gluten of wheat, etc.

*Fats:** Are stored as fat; e. g., fat of meat, butter, olive oil, oils of corn, wheat, etc.

*Carbohydrates:** Are transformed into fat; e. g., sugars, starches, etc.

Mineral matters (ash): Share in forming bone, assist in digestion; e. g., phosphates of lime, etc.; potash, soda, etc.

*All serve as building material and energy-producers.

[23]

All ingredients are necessary. If there is a shortage of mineral elements, the body quickly goes into disintegration.

Protein is what flesh is built from. It can be procured from all flesh of animals except fat. Grains furnish protein, and no doubt the body has power to synthesize protein from simple foods. All herbivora have the power to build flesh from grass. Our teaching leads us to think that without meat, eggs, or grain we cannot build muscle. Because of this idea or belief, there has grown up the very dangerous habit of eating too much meat and grain. As a consequence, nearly the whole human family is toxin-poisoned.

We have, when badly toxin-poisoned, lost the power to build protein out of the elemental foods—simple foods—such as fresh fruit, the succulent vegetables, and vegetable salads.

THE EVILS OF NEGLECTING TO EAT FRUIT AND SALAD

The continual eating of meat, bread, potatoes, etc., to the neglect of fresh, uncooked fruit and vegetables, is to disturb the distribution of the fluids of the body. The kidneys are over-worked, the bowels become constipated, the eyesight becomes perverted because of a change in the axis of the eye, eye-strain follows, and nervous derangements develop. Instead of correcting the errors of eating, glasses are fitted, and the victim of wrong eating is allowed to build other diseases.

Constipation, k i d n e y diseases, coughs, colds, bronchial, lung, and skin affections, are common to those who confine their eating to foods deprived of their watery elements, and who substitute coffee, tea, water, etc. Water, and the usual substitutes, fail to keep up elimination, and resulting autotoxemia develops from retention of excretions. These facts should compel all rational people to eat less so-called staple foods and more of fresh fruit and vegetable salads, and certainly to stop water-logging the body by drinking water*

SUSPENSION OF THE USE OF STAPLE FOODS

When the staple foods are given up, and the fruit and succulent vegetables are substituted, elimination begins. and will continue until the body is freed from retained debris. Weight is lost, and because of a suspension of

---

*Drinking water either water-logs the body or causes polyuria—excessive urination.

stimulating foods, and the elimination of retained toxins, the patient complains of a feeling of weakness. It is the same kind of weakness that takes hold of those who stop the use of alcohol, morphine, and other drugs. It will continue until the body is readjusted—reconstructed. Even professional men, who should know better, will declare to those perambulating, excretory depositories "You are starving to death! You need to eat good, nourishing food." Eating "good, nourishing food" is exactly what every toxin-poisoned—every sick—person has been doing; and there is no hope of recovery until "good, nourishing food" is supplanted by the simple fruits and vegetables.

LOSS OF FLESH AND ITS MEANING

When "good, nourishing" food is suspended to give nature a chance to throw off disease, the patient grows thinner. The fruits and salads act as eliminants, and the weight will run down until the house—the body—is cleaned; then there will be an increase in weight without an increase of the amount of food taken over the amount that permitted the decrease. Where the body is burdened with flesh, dropsy, and accumulated debris generally, there will be very rapid elimination, starting at once on the adoption of a fast. Such treatment should be watched by a competent physician; for cases have been known to collapse very suddenly after several days' fast.

To pass from a state in which staple foods have been eaten to the exclusion of fresh fruit and vegetables, until the patient is suffering from various affections superinduced by toxin poisoning, to a state freed from food poisoning and established on a rational food basis, takes time, and the transition cannot be made without more or less pain or discomfort.

CARBOHYDRATES (STARCH AND SUGAR)

These are the heat-producers. All the grains, potatoes, dry beans and peas furnish not only starch, but protein also.

These are the force foods, and in their entire state they are hard to digest by those who are seeking health, because of disease. Many sick people are injured and made into more confirmed invalids because of coarse eating. These are the people who are troubled greatly with gas in the bowels. Those troubled in this way should eat very lightly until they have recovered from this very disagreeable symptom. The starch-poisoned are hard to make comfortable without a fast, and many such patients complain bitterly of being so very weak without food.

Fats furnish energy—more, pound for pound, than starch and sugar. Sugar, however, yields energy more quickly.

The mineral elements are necessary for building purposes. The phosphatic salts are necessary for keeping the various tissues intact. Often these elements are lost because they are washed out of the body through the kidneys by the water-drinking habit, along with the eating of staple foods to the exclusion of fresh fruit and vegetables.

———◆———

In spite of allopathic medicines, all the chronic diseases of the last hundred years are with us.—Eli G. Jones, M.D.

• • •

Medicine is a science of guessing. —Dr. Abercrombie, F.R.C.P., Edinburgh.

General Outline for Menus

Every Other Day

BREAKFAST

Fruit

DINNER

Soup

(See page 58)

Meat

(See List 1, page 49)

Two Vegetables

(See List 3, page 49)

Salad

(See page 58)

SUPPER

Fresh fruit

Starch

(See List 4, page 50)

Every Alternate Day

BREAKFAST

Fruit

DINNER

Soup

(See page 58)

Starchy food carrying protein

(See List 2, page 49)

Two vegetables

(See List 3, page 49)

Any fresh fruit

SUPPER

Fresh fruit

Starch

(See List 4, page 50)

[29]

With the foregoing outlines, any housewife can select the proper combinations from the foods recommended by Dr. Tilden to be eaten together.

The evening meal of fruit and starch from List 4 (page 50) may be varied, taking one of the so-called desserts from List 5 (page 50) together with fruit. Such combinations are demonstrated in the specimen menus following.

———◆———

The popular medical system is a most uncertain and unsatisfactory system. It has neither philosophy nor common-sense to commend it to confidence. — Dr. Evans, F.R.C.P., London.

* * *

Correct diagnosis in many important diseases falls below fifty per cent in recognition, and in some below twenty-five per cent.—Hoerst Oertel, M.D., (Russell Sage Institute of Pathology).

* * *

Of all known sciences, none has been more unstable, confused, and contradictory in doctrine than medicine.—J. Rhodes Buchanan, M.D., Boston.

[30]

Specimen Menus for Winter Use

Monday—

BREAKFAST

Fresh fruit, with raisins, dates, or figs

DINNER

Tomato soup*

Salad

Lamb stew

Canned peas, parsnips

SUPPER

Fresh fruit

Toasted baking-powder biscuits

Tuesday—

BREAKFAST

Fresh fruit, with raisins, dates, or figs

DINNER

Vegetable soup

Grapefruit

Hubbard squash

Canned corn, turnips

SUPPER

Apple pie

Fruit or milk

*Those who are decidedly constipated; or those with too much saliva, troubled with ptyalism, gastic catarrh, should not eat soup of any kind.

[31]

Wednesday—

BREAKFAST

Canned fruit, with raisins, dates,
or figs

DINNER

Roast Pork*

Stewed or baked apples

Salad or grapefruit

Stewed tomatoes, spinach

SUPPER

Rice with cream, half milk

Fresh fruit

Thursday—

BREAKFAST

Fresh fruit, with raisins, dates, or figs

DINNER

Vegetable soup

Hominy

Cabbage, rutabagas

Grapefruit

SUPPER

Baked custard or ice cream

Cake

*Pork, sausage, and fat fish require much fruit acid to aid digestion. Lemon should be used freely. In the absence of lemon or acid fruit, use cider vinegar.

Friday—

Fresh fruit, with raisins, dates, or figs

Tomato soup

Fish

String beans, stewed onions

Salad

Oatmeal, dressed with milk, half cream

Fresh fruit

Saturday—

Fresh fruit, with raisins, dates, or figs

Vegetable soup

Baked beans*

Parsnips, carrots

Grapefruit

Canned pineapple

Cottage or cream cheese

*Beans, pork, and fat fish are very taxing on the stomach. The best way to eat them is with a good-sized combination salad, dressed with salt, olive oil, and plenty of lemon—Nothing else.

Sunday—

BREAKFAST

Canned fruit, with raisins, dates,
or figs

DINNER

Tomato soup

Celery and olives

Roast fowl or game

Jelly or preserves

Salad

String beans, stewed tomatoes

Fruit pie or ice cream

SUPPER

Plain cake

Fresh fruit

———◆———

Ninety per cent of my fellow-practitioners are quacks. — Dr. Schweninger, Physician to Bismarck.

• • •

The arrival of a clown in town is worth more than the arrival of twenty medical quacks with drugs. —Prof. Sydenham, noted English Physician.

• • •

It is the best physician who gives the least medicine. Drug physicians are quacks. — Benjamin Franklin Philosopher.

[34]

Special Menus for Summer Use

Monday—

BREAKFAST
Fresh fruit

DINNER
Celery soup*
Broiled steak
Salad
Beets, spinach

SUPPER
Fresh fruit
Toasted biscuit

Tuesday—

BREAKFAST
Fresh fruit

DINNER
Vegetable soup
Baked potatoes
Salad
String beans, stewed onions

SUPPER
Ice-cream
Cake

(*See footnote, page 61)

Wednesday—

BREAKFAST
Fresh fruit

DINNER
Two poached eggs
Salad
Green peas, sweet corn

SUPPER
Fresh fruit
Sponge cake

Thursday—

BREAKFAST
Fresh fruit

DINNER
Potato soup
Corn bread
Cauliflower, asparagus
Salad

SUPPER
Fresh fruit
Ice-cream

[36]

Friday—

Fresh fruit or cantaloupe

Broiled fish
Salad
Kohlrabi, beets

Fresh fruit
Triscuit or toasted bread

Saturday—

Fresh fruit

Vegetable soup
Macaroni
Sweet corn, stewed celery
Salad

Corn bread, butter and
Milk or fruit

[37]

Sunday—

BREAKFAST

Fresh fruit

DINNER

Tomato soup

Celery, olives

Chicken

Jelly or preserves

Asparagus, spinach

Salad

Fruit Jello or ices

SUPPER

Fresh fruit

Ice-cream or watermelon alone

The following menus are intended for people leading very active lives—mechanics, farmers, etc.:

Monday—

Corn bread, butter
Apples or milk*

Tomato soup
Corn beef and cabbage
Salad
Canned corn, carrots

Oatmeal
Fresh fruit

Tuesday—

Toasted biscuit
Honey

Potato soup
Baked potatoes
Salad
Turnips, sweet corn

Fresh fruit
Cottage or cream cheese

*Those who are troubled with catarrh, hay fever, or constipation, should not use milk.

Wednesday—

BREAKFAST

Buckwheat cakes

Country sausage

DINNER

Tomato soup

Bacon and eggs

Salad

Spinach, cauliflower

SUPPER

Custard

Plain cake

Thursday—

BREAKFAST

Baking-powder biscuit

Bacon

Fruit

DINNER

Vegetable soup

Macaroni

Salad

Stewed onions, carrots and peas

SUPPER

Apple pie

Cheese

Fresh fruit

Friday—

Corn bread, butter
Honey
Fresh fruit

DINNER
Vegetable soup
Roast pork, baked apples
Grapefruit
Stewed tomatoes, parsnips

SUPPER
Fresh fruit

Saturday—

BREAKFAST
Muffins, butter
Fruit

DINNER
Baked beans
Salad
Turnips, canned corn

SUPPER
Cottage cheese
Fresh fruit

Sunday—

Waffles, honey
Fresh fruit

Tomato soup
Olives, celery
Roast Chicken
Jelly
Salad
String beans, beets
Ice-cream

Fresh fruit
Cake

Menus for School Children

Monday—

BREAKFAST

Fresh biscuit, butter,
Honey
Milk

LUNCH

Toasted bread, butter,
Apples

DINNER

Poached eggs
Salad
Turnips, spinach

Tuesday—

BREAKFAST

Oatmeal mush, salt, butter
Glass of milk

LUNCH

Plain cake
Fresh fruit

DINNER

Baked potato
Salad
Carrots, corn

[43]

Wednesday—

BREAKFAST
Corn bread, butter
Milk

LUNCH
Graham crackers
Fruit

DINNER
Stewed lamb
Grapefruit
Peas, stewed tomatoes

Thursday—

BREAKFAST
Baked apples, raisins
Milk

LUNCH
Toasted biscuit
Fresh fruit

DINNER
Rice
Salad
Spinach, stewed onions

Friday—

Muffins, butter
Milk

LUNCH
Ginger bread
Fresh fruit

DINNER
Fish
Grapefruit
Greens, cauliflower

Saturday—

BREAKFAST
Cream of Wheat
Fresh fruit

LUNCH
Pie, cheese,
Milk

DINNER
Baked beans
Salad
String beans, cabbage

[45]

Sunday—

BREAKFAST

Pancakes, butter, maple syrup

Milk

DINNER

Chicken

Salad

Jelly

Turnips, peas

Fruit Jello

SUPPER

Ice-cream

Cake

A Few Additions for Variety's Sake

(1) Occasionally those in perfect health may take ice-cream, ices, prune-whip, Jello, fruit pie, cake, or custard as dessert for dinner.

(2) Tapioca pudding, rice pudding, or any other of the starchy puddings may be used with fruit for the evening meal.

(3) If it is impossible to get material for the salad, use cold slaw (see page 59 for recipe) or grapefruit.

(4) Bannanas, being one of the hardest fruits to digest, should be taken alone for breakfast or lunch. The same applies to watermelon, cantaloupe, or any other melon in season. Those in perfect health may mix all kinds of foods—make all kinds of conglomerations—as long as health lasts; but when digestive power is once broken, no other food should be eaten with melons. Those troubled with indigestion should not begin a breakfast with cantaloupe—eat the melon without other food.

[47]

(5) If desired, the dinner may be served in the evening, and the menus suggested for the evening meal may be used for the lunch at noon.

(6) Left-over meat may be ground up and added to vegetable soup just before serving. This dish should then be used in place of other meat in a dinner.

———◆———

The distinction between the quack doctor and the qualified one is merely that the latter is allowed to sign death certificates, for which both sorts have equal occasion.—Bernard Shaw.

* * *

I sincerely believe that the un-biased opinion of most medical men of sound mind and long medical experience is that the amount of death and disaster in the world would be less than it now is if all disease were left to itself.—J. Bigelow, M.D. in Rational Medicine.

* * *

The doctor never advertises his incompetency by admitting his mistakes, but hides his incompetency and mistakes by saying the patient died from unforseen complications. —Journal American Medical Association.

List 1

MEAT, OR ITS PROTEIN EQUIVALENT

(For dinner use only.)

Lamb, fowl, fish, eggs, mutton, game, sweetbreads, calves' liver, sausage, oysters or other sea food, beef, veal, pork, milk, buttermilk, cheese, nuts, sardines or other canned fish, smoked or cured meats.

List 2

STARCHY FOODS CARRYING PROTEIN

(Substitutes for meat.)

Sweet potatoes, Irish potatoes, hominy, Hubbard squash, macaroni, spaghetti, baked beans, any dry beans or peas, rice, corn bread, whole-wheat bread, rye bread.

List 3

NON-STARCHY VEGETABLES

Carrots, beet tops, beets, spinach, parsnips, cauliflower, turnips, kohlrabi, cabbage, kale, stewed celery, corn, peas, green beans, asparagus, rutabagas, oyster plant, egg plant, dandelion, onions, summer squash, salsify, okra, Brussels sprouts, tomatoes, endive, chard.

List 4

DECIDEDLY STARCHY FOODS

(For use at evening lunch)

Baking-powder biscuit (fresh or toasted), muffins, Shredded Wheat, Triscuit, Puffed Wheat, Puffed Rice, or any flake foods, Royal Toast crackers, zwieback, Cream of Wheat, Rolled Oats, Farina, rice, or any of the cereal breakfast foods.

List 5

SO-CALLED DESSERTS*

(For use as suggested for lunch or occasionally as dessert)

Ice-cream, ices, tapioca pudding, rice pudding, custard, fruit pies, prune-whip, jello.

*Desserts cause overeating, and for this reason are objectionable. Pie and a glass of milk, or cake and milk or ice-cream, for lunch, but not as dessert, will do little harm to healthy people.

* * *

If medicine is to remain a profession, this competition for money must cease.—Richard C. Cabot, Chief Medical Staff, Massachusetts General Hospital (from Literary Digest.)

A Few Don'ts

(1) It is best not to eat cooked fruit (sugared and creamed), jellies, preserves, butters, marmalades, etc., with any kind of bread, toast, cereals, or starch in any form.

(2) Fresh fruits may be eaten with starchy foods, but it is best to eat only well-ripened and sweet or subacid fruits. When there is great irritation of the stomach, fruit and starch should not be eaten together. Indeed, the use of starchy foods, such as grain and potatoes, should be suspended until the irritation subsides.

(3) Canned goods are not recommended except where it is impossible to get fresh food. The same holds good for smoked and cured meats, with the exception of a little bacon, which may be used with starchy foods, inasmuch as it is mostly fat, but not proteid as other meats.

(4) If dependable health is desired, do not eat anything between meals, and do not eat without a keen relish— and *not then, unless absolute comfort*

has been experienced since the previous meal. (See rules, page 53.)

(5) If constipated, do not drink anything between meals nor at meal-time. If the bowels are regular and can be depended upon to move daily, water, teakettle tea, or cereal coffee may be used at meal-time. Cold water may be used at meal-time, but not within four hours after leaving the table. If thirst is driving, warm water may be taken.

(6) Stewed tomatoes cause discomfort when eaten with starchy foods. Raw tomatoes **may be taken** with starch.

———◆———

The function of the tonsil is unknown, and, therefore, these organs should not be removed.—John McKenzie, Professor in John Hopkins University. (By the way, he was a throat specialist.—J.H.T.)

* * *

Back of disease lies a cause, and the cause no drug can reach.—S. Weir Mitchell, M.D.

The Four Tilden Rules

Rule No. 1: Never eat unless comfortable in mind and body from the previous meal—or meal-time.

Rule No. 2: Never eat without desire and a keen relish for the plainest and simplest foods; and not then, if to do so will cause the breaking of the first rule.

Rule No. 3: Avoid overeating. This is best accomplished by observing Rule No. 4.

Rule No. 4: Thoroughly masticate and insalivate all foods.

Proper Cooking

VEGETABLES

Vegetables should be prepared and put to cook in just enough water to prevent burning. When properly cooked, the water should be practically all boiled away. What water remains should be a rich juice and should be served with the vegetables. Positively no seasoning is to be added to any food until served; then each person should season to suit himself, with salt, and butter or cream. Do not use flour or starch dressings, or so-called cream dressings. The cooking-vessel should have a tight-fitting cover. A double boiler may often be used to advantage; it minimizes the danger of burning. Steam cooking is an ideal way, and the fireless cooking is said to give satisfaction. When the double boiler is used, little, if any, water is needed. The more nearly vegetables are cooked in their own juice, the better. Any two vegetables may be cooked together, but vegetables should not be cooked with meat.

Dry Beans and Peas—These two foods are injured by the practice of soaking overnight, and then throwing off the water in which they were soaked and cooking in fresh water. In soaking, the soda is thrown off with the water, and the alkaline potentiality of the food is destroyed. These two starchy foods should be soaked overnight and cooked in the water in which they were soaked. No seasoning should be added until served, then butter and salt may be added to taste.

MEATS

Meats should never be fried. Pot-roasting is well suited for small families. Put the roast to cook in a small amount of cold water after having seared it well on all sides. Allow it to come to the boiling-point very slowly; then turn the gas down to the simmering-point. Just enough water should be used so that, when the meat is tender, it will all be evaporated. If, by mistake too much water has been used, the fluid may be used for soup, or to dress the cooked vegetables in place of butter or cream.

Steaks and Chops should be broiled. Sear the meat well on both sides, very quickly; then finish the cooking with enough heat to cook the inside of the meat without hardening the albumin.

In broiling, the object is to sacrifice the outside of the meat—harden the albumin of the surface of the meat—but keep the inside soft and juicy.

Fish should be washed and dried; then laid on a greased paper in a baking-pan. Bake until tender, and dress with salt, lemon juice, and butter if the fish is not fat.

Jacket Roasting.—Roasting in a jacket is a good way to prevent the meat from drying out. Make a batter of flour and water. The batter should be stiff enough to coat the meat well. After giving the prospective roast a thorough coating, wrap paper with another layer of the batter. Roast the regulation time, adding a little extra on account of the jacket. When done, the jacket may be split down the middle and the meat lifted out.

Any meat may be cooked in this way; veal, beef, mutton, fowl, or pork. Pork is especially fine when thus cooked.

Round Steak.—Round steak—the cheapest of steaks—cooked as follows is quite palatable: Put into a very hot frying-pan and sear thoroughly; then allow it to stew by adding a small

[56]

amount of cold water. The cooking, until the meat is tender, should be by a simmering heat rather than by hard boiling. When tender, take up on a hot plate, cover, and place in a warming-oven.

———◆———

Most of the colic cures and medicines for summer sicknesses contain some fairly powerful narcotic.—Woods Hutchinson, M.D., New York American, June 30. (There are legions in Heaven prematurely because of it.—J.H.T.)

* * *

The whole theory of vaccination and serum is erroneous; for, although by their use we may obtain freedom from one disease, it lays us liable to others, especially tuberculosis.—Lieut. C. E. Woodruff, U. S. Army.

* * *

Diseases have increased in proportion as medical men have increased.—Dr. Abernathy, M. D., London.

A Few Tilden Receipes

TILDEN COMBINATION SALAD

Lettuce, tomatoes, cucumbers, a small bit of onion. Dress with salt, olive oil, and lemon juice.

Lettuce, celery, canned tomatoes, or fruit, such as apples and grapes. Dressing the same as above.

VEGETABLE SOUP

Turnip, carrot, spinach, celery, cabbage, onion, green corn, peas, beans, potato. Run any five of the above vegetables through a vegetable mill, and cook in enough water to keep from burning. When thoroughly cooked add enough milk to make the desired amount of soup. Add salt and butter after serving. Any left-over vegetables may be used in preparing this soup. Oyster plant, left-over, stewed or baked beans, or cold potatoes may be used. If it is to be served with meat meal, a little meat broth may be added.

CREAM-OF-TOMATO SOUP

1 pint tomatoes, strained   1 cup milk
1 cup cream

Put tomatoes in double boiler and, when near boiling-point, add one-half teaspoon of soda. Add milk and cream (hot) to tomatoes, and season with salt and pepper; or drop cream and add one cup of broth.

COLD SLAW.

After cabbage has been thoroughly cooled in cold water, cut fine. Dress with lemon juice, cream, either sweet or sour, and a very little salt.

BAKED PORK AND BEANS

The beans should be put to soak the night before they are to be served. When they are put to cook the next morning, the same water should be used in which they have been soaked. Enough more water should be added to just come to the top of the beans. Allow to cook until all the water is cooked away, and then put into a baking-pan with a very small amount of water. Add more in small amounts as necessary.

When thoroughly cooked, the fire on the oven should be turned very low. Take a strip or two of bacon and put to stew in a small amount of water, after having cut it into small pieces. When tender, pour the juice and the pieces of bacon over the beans—about twenty minutes before serving time— and allow to stand until taken up.

TILDEN BISCUIT

1 quart flour

Salt sufficient

1 heaping teaspoon baking powder*

2 tablespoons melted butter

Milk sufficient to make soft dough

*Schilling's Baking Powder is reliable.

Rub the baking-powder, salt, butter, and flour together. Add milk, and manipulate rapidly into a soft dough. Biscuit dough should be teased, rather than rolled, into a sheet about one-half inch thick. Cut into strips one and one-half inches wide. Place in baking-pan. Have oven at a baking temperature, and get dough into oven as quickly as possible.

CORN-MEAL MUFFINS

½ cup corn meal
½ cup white flour
1 egg well beaten
1 teaspoon baking-powder
½ cup sweet milk
1 teaspoon melted butter

Mix flour and baking-powder with salt. Add milk, beaten egg, and melted butter. This makes six.

CEREALS

In cooking oatmeal, or any of the breakfast cereals, use about one part of the cereal to five parts of water. Cook until the mixture has reached the consistency of mush. Then dress with salt, and butter, or salt and cream—no sugar.

MACARONI

Macaroni should be kept boiling constantly in a large amount of water. When tender, drain off water and, after placing in colander, allow cold water to run through it. Just before serving, add salt and butter or a little cream, no cheese or tomato dressing.

CLABBER BUTTERMILK

Pour fresh, clean milk into a deep dish, and allow to stand until clabbered as thick as baked custard. Then chill, and beat with an egg-beater thoroughly, incorporating as much air as possible.

------◆------

If, in diptheria, the bacillus is not found, the illness is renamed by the doctors as something else.—Encyclopedia Britannica.

• • •

Consumption is caused by Peruvian bark.—Dr. Stabi, M.D.

Peruvian bark is an effectual cure for consumption.—Dr. Martin, M.D.

• • •

Probably seventy-five percent of the people who come to us would get well in spite of what we do for them.—Geo. H. Matson, M.D., Secretary Ohio State Medical Board, in A. M. A. Bulletin No. 15. (Dr. Matson is the moving spirit in attempts to exterminate the drugless healers in Ohio.)

Chapter II.
What is Health?

Health is a state of the body where c o m f o r t reigns supreme. Health means the absence of all the disagreeable appearances of disease. The skin is clear, the eyes are bright, the body is erect, the mind is alert, and the emotions are under control. The healthy —those in full possession of health— do not have headache, toothache, backache, tic douloureux (painful twitching) leg-ache, that dreadful tired feeling, short breath. Indeed, those in health have no discomforts. The desire for food, when normal, is never urgent—compelling. If food is not forthcoming, there is not a feeling of great discomfort, expressed differently by different people, such as: "I shall famish if I do not eat; I shall faint; I'm so weak that I shall die unless I can get my dinner; I have a dreadful all-gone feeling, and must eat to relieve it." Healthy, normal people are not compelled to rush the growler —any old growler, from absinthe to water—or famish—die of thirst.

Where there is a disease-provoking habit established, we hear such remarks as: "I shall have headache if I do not get my coffee; my head is splitting because I did not get my coffee, my tea, my cocoa, my lunch." Those who regularly overeat, before they admit that they are sick, or have become regular visitors to the doctor shops—before they have established the doctoring habit — will be heard complaining of nervousness, sleepless nights, itching of the surface of the b o d y , prickling sensations, hives, herpes (cold sores), eczema, and other skin symptoms; a feeling of tension in the legs, and a desire to move them frequently, w i t h o u t relief when moved; restlessness, which moving about or changing position does not relieve.

Cough is one of the early symptoms of overeating or haphazard eating. This is the cough that annoys in public places, and which is heard at churches, theatres, and gatherings of various kinds. Ṣore throat, tonsilitis, or quinsy is in constant attendance on imprudent eating by many people.

Enlarged tonsils, adenoids, polypi, spurs (bony growths) chronic rhinitis, and hay-fever are throat and nose affections of nicotinites, bibbers, and the glutted.

Irregular bowels, constipation, and all the dire consequences of toxin poisoning which are necessary resultants of gastro-intestinal indigestion from overeating, are symptoms that trouble the masses. From this source the surgeon gets most of his excuses for operating—for removing organs which are affected by the general toxemia, but which for the most part are only symptoms, and which, when removed, leave the disease behind.

Persistent overindulgence at the table causes gastro-intestinal indigestion; catarrh and constipation follow; and this furnishes the basis or cause, directly or indirectly, of all the sickness—so called diseases—and crime calendared.

A FEW OF THE DISEASES INCIDENT TO DAILY LIFE

Gas in the bowels, irregular movements—free movements, even a diarrhea for two or three days, followed with constipation requiring cathartics or enemas—are quite common affections. If the stools are watched, much mucous (catarrhal secretion) will be seen passing with the feces. In severe constipation the feces are dessicated into scybala (hard, lumpy formations). These have a grayish, glassy appearance. When constipated feces have this appearance, it indicates colitis (catarrh of the large intestine). The rectum is often involved. The symptoms indicating this involvement are much catarrhal discharge—not necessarily connected with the hard fecal lumps, but passing unmixed, accompanied with bearing down, a feeling that the evacuation is not complete, but which discomfort often gradually passes away without any further evacuation. Gradually there develops a hemorrhoidal state of the mucous membrane, with more or less hemorrhage or bleeding at each evacuation. In time prolapsus, or a rolling-out of a large fold of mucous membrane and submucous tissue, develops which is very annoying. If the bowel movement takes place in the morning, the tendency will be for the prolapsus to remain out all day, making it necessary to replace it often to get relief. The eating of starches and sweets increases this affection. Surgery offers, for cure, removal of pile tumors, or the removal of the part of the rectal mucous membrane that rolls out and annoys. The adoption of moderate eating and daily exercise will overcome piles and prolapsus. Colitis or constipation can be overcome if the victim of this disease will modify his style of living.

THE AFFECTIONS LEADING TO POPULAR OPERATIONS

The colitis above referred to is caused by intestinal decomposition. Gas is an almost constant symptom. When the colitis is severe, the bowel is sensitive, and the gas distention brings on much discomfort. When the distention is acute and located in the region of the appendix, the diagnosis is too often appendicitis, and much too often the treatment is an operation. It is obvious that, if the colitis continues, pain must be duplicated, and the diagnosis the next time may be disease of the right ovary. Another operation is recommended—this time for the removal of the ovary—and, of course, is consented to. After the ovary is removed, the colitis, indigestion, and gas distention remain, with the accompanying discomfort, which is now attributed to adhesions by the surgeons. An operation for breaking up adhesions is consented to. After its performance the colitis, intestinal indigestion, and gas distention continue, with increasing discomfort, which from the first was sensitiveness to pressure when the distention was least, discomfort when gas was moderate, but much pain, or excruciating suffering, when the gas distention was greatest.

At this stage the patient has a very large sick habit developed; besides, resistance is broken, and the patient suffers in mind as well as body. For the suffering that develops at this stage, surgery may offer drainage of the gall-bladder, removal of the gall-bladder, removal of the remaining reproductive organs, operations on kidneys, or re-re-re-operations for breaking up adhesions, until the patient dies from exhaustion, or septic poisoning, as did a governor of one of the northern states a few years ago.

From the beginning to the end of this life-picture, representing the supreme inefficiency of modern medical and surgical science, there has been interpolated scientific diagnosis galore: blood tests, X-ray pictures, microscopic findings, consultations, change of climate, and special seances with all the specialists belonging to the profession.

Is the above word-picture a pipe-dream? Reason and faith in an honorable profession declare that it must be. And reason would stand confirmed in its opinion, if thousands of mutilated—vandalized—victims of the Moloch of surgery did not grace our country today. They are to be found in ever city, and in about every hamlet. All may not register up to the full quota of operations; but if they do not, it is because they have not had time, or they have not the price, or have not found some professional man needing surgical experience.

COULD BE AVOIDED

All this horrid vandalism could be avoided if people were willing to believe that all of their sufferings are brought on them by breaking the laws of health—that disease is health struggling under a handicap. If this truth could become a part of humanity, and be acted upon wisely—namely, remove the cause as soon as discovered—we should soon evolve a race of normal human beings instead of, as we see now, a race of invalids.

[68]

SHOULD PEOPLE BE KEPT IN IGNORANCE OF DISEASE?

There is quite a popular belief that lay people should not read about disease. That must, of course, depend on what they read. The same can, with as much truth, be said of every form of reading. There is bad and good reading on every subject, there is good and bad in all books—yes, even in good books—and people should read much, that they may learn to judge of the good and the bad. People who are prejudiced, and carry into their reading preconceptions, of course will finish as they begin. They cultivate prejudice, which in time bars truth, shuts them out forever from the best in life, and sends them to a premature grave. The simple, open mind is the only one that attracts truth; wise and "sufficient unto the day" drives real wisdom away.

To watch for symptoms is not good; neither is it necessary, if a proper understanding of their import is well in mind. To illustrate: A pain in the right lower abdominal region in these days of thinking in the language of disease and surgery, may suggest to the patient appendicitis. If he consults a physician who agree with him, an operation may be forthcoming. And all the excuse for operating is fear on the part of the patient, and a hyper-willingness to operate on the part of the surgeon; the cause being gas pressure from indigestion, colitis, or constipation. The patient should know that constipation is liable to cause pain in the lower bowels. If there is distention of an inflamed colon, from gas, pain is sure to be present; there is usually constipation, and the hardened feces, as well as the gas, cause pain. An enema of warm water will generally relieve the pain. When appendicitis has been subjected to malpractice and rough bimanual manipulation, it may be necessary to operate to save life.

IN REGARD TO OPERATING

Wait! Don't be in a hurry to have an operation! If it is appendicitis, the best treatment is to keep in bed, and refuse to eat or drink anything until comfortable. Water may be taken at pleasure, after the nausea has passed, but no food until the bowels have moved and complete comfort is restored. One enema every night until the bowels move from above the abscess, which will happen as soon as the abscess breaks into the bowel, which it will do if not trifled with by frequent examinations. The pressure made by doctors in examining these cases often ruptures the abscess and forces a speedy operation. When not roughly handled, these abscesses will not rupture other than into the bowel —the natural outlet.

Many people think they have heart disease because the heart is made to palpitate from indigestion. If rapid heart action, with palpitation, follows a dinner, it means overeating, or perhaps a little indigestion which will pass off. If much fat, or fatty foods, be eaten, the juice of a lemon should help the stomach to digest; if much starch has been eaten, then the heart palpitation and oppression — short breath—can be relieved with bi-carbonate of soda (baking soda). The prudent will modify their eating and end such discomforts.

A sensitive spot over the ribs will often be thought lung disease. If the spot is sensitive to touch, it is intercostal (between-the-ribs) rheumatism and has nothing to do with the lungs.

A lump in the breast will often be mistaken for cancer. Remember that these lumps are more often enlarged

[71]

glands, accompanying menstruation, and are caused by imprudent eating and constipation. It is a crime to cut such breasts off.

It is worth while to know that pneumonia cannot develop in any person who is not constipated and who is prudent in eating.

It is worth much to know that it takes years of imprudence in eating, abuse and neglect of the body to develop tuberculosis in those who are of the tubercular diathesis—with an in herited tendency to take on the disease. If germs caused the disease, there would be no human being left on earth to tell the story.

The same is true of all the derangements of the body. Then why is teaching a popular knowledge of those facts so very unwise? Is it unwise to have laymen understand law—understand that to break certain laws of city, state, or nation will bring on punishment? Because of the knowledge, will they be more likely to break the law? Is it a fact that to know law is to break it? Certainly this is a fool's reasoning.

To know that discomforts of all kinds come from wrong living is to arm the one possessed of such knowledge with self-protection. To know the cause of a pain is to know the remedy. The average human being, when sick, is a helpless victim of a commercialized medical profession, and one that is educated out of all commonsense. People are being very wisely—scientifically—deprived of life.

If tobacco is the cause of an overworked heart, then to stop the use of it will effect a cure. Certainly it is foolish to further weaken the organ by taking heart stimulants. If it is coffee, or tea, or alcoholics that cause the discomfort, then the cure must be to stop the toxin that causes it. Yes, any intoxicant is a toxin—it may be an animal or vegetable alkaloid. The animal alkaloid is usually called ptomaine.

If it is a fact that sickness is the rule, and health the exception, in our civilization, and that no one really dies of old age, does it not stand to reason that something is radically wrong with our manner of living? As man is a digestive and reproductive apparatus, it is obvious to the discerning and reflective that his derangements must be abuse of digestion and the function of reproduction. To learn the causes of perverted functioning—cause of disease—the subject of disease must be studied in their relation to their building-up and their tearing-down processes. Certainly it stands to reason that these functions must be abused—over-used; and in what way, it is necessary to discover; for then the correcting — the curing — may be in keeping with the cause.

————◆————

If we arrive at a correct diagnosis in only fifty per cent, are we not quacks to the extent of the other fifty per cent in diagnosing and giving treatment.—Richard Cabot, Chief Medical Staff, Massachusetts General Hospital.

• • •

The germ theory of disease is based upon the misconception that germs are the cause instead of being the effect of the disease.—Lieut. C. E. Woodruff, U. S. Army.

• • •

If it is legal to leave health regulations to doctors, why should we not leave the regulation of burglary to burglars?—C. R. Lipman, quoting Life.

Chapter III

The First Cause of the Cause of All Diseases

The primary cause of the cause (autotoxemia) of all diseases is *gastro-intestinal fermentation and decomposition*. Cold, coryza, influenza, la grippe, tonsilitis, bronchitis, pneumonia, gastritis, are all one and the same, varying in local manifestations and intensity, but all resting on the one base —namely, gastric fermentation. If eating be discontinued, these various manifestations will end with the ending of the fermentation. Where the gastric fermentation is continued by improper eating day after day, and becomes chronic, the manifestations will be gastritis, with all the different forms of so-called dyspepsia, dilation of the stomach, ulceration, pyloric obstructions, and cancer. Duodenal ulcer, catarrh of the gall-duct, gall-bladder, and pancreatic duct, and pancreatitis, are all simply extension of gastritis—chronic gastric fermentation.

When the fermentation extends to the intestine, the symptoms of catarrhal inflammation which it produces are named, according to locality: intestinal catarrh, gastro-enteritis, colitis, appendicits, diarrhea, constipation, proctitis, and many other well-known diseases unnecessary to mention, which are collateral to the intestine and connected therewith by the lymphatic, blood, and nervous systems.

The two most pronounced symptoms of the many that develop because of gastro-intestinal fermentation are gastritis and colitis. The gastric symptoms are named above, beginning with colds and coryza or catarrh. Colitis is known by its two most frequent symptoms—diarrhea and constipation.

Where gastritis and colitis are established, acidosis becomes constitutional in the former, and in the latter, toxemia. Between the two sources we have chronic *auto-intoxication* or *auto-toxemia*—THE CAUSE of all the auto-generated diseases known to medical science and recorded in nomenclature.

There is not a disease that cannot be traced to the gastro-intestinal tract as the source of its origin—or, if not of its origin, then to its continuance.

This statement will appear so extravagant that perhaps the rank and file of medical men will turn from it with a feeling of pity or disgust—or maybe without even that much attention; with pity, that a man should be busy in a profession for forty-six years and know no more; or with disgust, because of the audacity of an ignoramus in obtruding his opinion on a wise medical world. No perturbance, however, will be felt because of either of these wise, or otherwise, conclusions. Instead, our purpose to perfect the application of these principles to the restoration of health will go on, and the enjoyment of seeing people get well, where the principles are worked out, will be compensation quite sufficient for all the scorn and ostracism, be they heaped to heaven by the representatives of a modern science of healing that is perfect in every detail except in healing.

Assuming that the theory of the cause of disease advanced above is correct, it behooves every man and woman, as well as every child of sufficient comprehension, to become mentally possessed of every suggestion contained in this little book, and to put it into practice. Certainly no harm can come to those who do so; and this is more than can be said of most of what is falsely named scientific *doctoring* and *immunization*.

Colds (Coryza)

Colds mean acute gastritis (indigestion). To cure them, stop eating, in order to empty the stomach; clear out the bowels with enemas.* Remember: "If you feed a cold, you will have to starve a fever." Stop eating until all symptoms have disappeared; then eat fruit the first day, and thereafter eat lightly until sensations (feelings) are perfectly normal. Those with the tuberculosis diathesis will never develop the disease, if eating be in keeping with the suggestions herein contained, and every cold taken be treated in this way.

Those of a gouty diathesis will never develop rheumatism, if all colds are controlled as above directed.

The same is true of the neurotic and all other diathesis (inherited tendencies).

*Enemas are to be used in emergencies only —in acute indigestion, typhoid fever, appendicitis, and always where there appears to be obstruction.

Colitis (Constipation)

Catarrhal inflamation of the colon is known by the name of colitis, Diarrhea and constipation are the two most pronounced symptoms. When constipation is established, there is always polyuria (too much activity of the kidneys). When there is diarrhea the fluids are diverted into the bowels, and the kidneys fail to receive their share of fluid, which in time will pervert the functioning of these organs.

The first and most necessary symptom to control in chronic constipation is the diversion of fluids to the kidneys. This can be done by stopping the drinking of water and all table beverages. The thirst must be suffered; for there is no other way to force nature to reestablish the lost function of secretion into the bowels. This is contrary to my former teaching, and the popular teaching of today, regarding water-drinking; but, to progress it is necessary to make changes, and I do so without apology. To take drugs for constipation is worse than useless, notwithstanding the fact that the universe has been searched for a physic, cathartic, aperient, or a laxative with which to regulate the bowels. But, alas! closely following on the heels of each *new eureka* has been heard the doleful sound of failure.

The enema habit usually follows the cathartic habit, with its inevitable confirmation of failure. Of course, the numerous devices for flooding the bowels do wash out accumulated debris; but *at no time are constipation and its cause cured*. The real cause must continue, and toxic infection must be endured until fatal disease of the various organs of the body develop unless the *usual cures* are supplanted by the inhibition of water and table beverages until secretions are established in the bowels.

Why should a search for a cure-all be crowned with success? Certainly guessing will not succeed in the medical profession any better than in other departments of human endeavor. Up to the present no special thought has been given to the real cause of constipation; hence the reason for the disgraceful failure of the profession in being able to give the advice necessary for a cure. When fluid diversion to the kidneys is controlled, every case of constipation that is not dependent on mechanical obstructions can be cured.

Bran and coarse bread are looked upon by many as wise and logical cures for the victims of the cathartic and enema habits. But, alas and alack! the cure is but a childish guess. Those who need a cure most are those who have least power to extract nourishment from such bread; and, as for raw bran, the raw starch in it adds to chronic gastro-intestinal fermentation, and the hull of the grain pricks the sensitive mucous membrane, causing more mucus to be thrown out and thereby inhibiting more and more an already retarded digestion. It is a remedy that has received no thought— it is simply an unwise guess.

Drinking Without Thirst

Why should one drink without thirst? Is this more sensible than eating without desire? Certainly it is necessary to discriminate between a normal thirst and an abnormal desire for fluid or water-drinking.

Where there is no overeating, or improper mixing of foods, or an excessive use of condiments, there will not be much, if any, thirst. Active exercise in hot weather, or work in super-

heated workshops—such as glass fac-
tories, machine shops, smelters, found-
ries, etc.—drives those thus engaged
to drink. Even in overheated places
workmen should use much self-control
and learn to eat in such a way as not
to build an abnormal desire for liquids.

Those who suffer from the heat of
summer are invariably those who eat
and drink too much.

Those working in superheated workshops, and who give way to thirst, soon
build a waterlogging habit. Of course,
disease and a general break-down must
follow.

Those working in moderate heat, as
out-of-doors in hot weather, will not
desire an excess of water, unless they
overeat, or eat too much condiment
with their food.

Impulsive people get the tarred end
of the stick every time. When one
of this temperament sees someone else
drink, he is seized with an impulse
to drink. The question of thirst is
not thought about; much less is a
thought given to the idea that water,
taken in excess, is disease-building.

Water-drinking, like the drinking of
alcoholics, is an unnecessary habit.
One drink, from a half to one hour
after a hearty meal, calls for another,

and then another, and still another, until indigestion follows. This habit, continued, will build chronic gastritis, which will end in dilation, ulcer, or cancer.

When thirst follows a dinner, it should not be indulged. If it is not, it will prove to be a demand, which, if not satisfied from without, by water-drinking, will be met in full from within, by the gastro-intestinal secretory glands pouring into the canal all the fluid necessary; and along with the fluid will be enough enzymic ferment to finish the digestion perfectly.

Rapid Eating

Bolting of food is aided by water-drinking and table beverages. The reward of disease is waiting for the food-bolter just a short distance ahead. If no fluid is taken while eating, or after the meal is finished, the eating may be done as rapidly as possible, and no harm can follow: for the thirst if endured, will be satisfied with the normal secretions, and the demand for fluid that was almost irresistible will pass away, leaving a feeling of general comfort; whereas, if the food is washed into the stomach, and drinking is indulged in after eating, a feeling of discomfort will be experienced.

When all the fruit, salad, and cooked succulent vegetables are eaten that should be eaten each day, and condiments are limited, there will be no need of drinking at meal-time, or between meals, when the drinking habit is over-come.

An excessive intake of fluids at meal-time, and between meals, certainly interferes with all secretions; and when there is not enough secretion in the mouth, stomach, and bowels, indigestion follows, with all its dire consequences.

If water-drinking is more or less injurious, it must be obvious to the discerning that tea, coffee, alcoholics, and soda-fountain drinks must also do harm, in proportion to their use. The occasional drinker will experience no harm, harm comes when habit is formed and interferes with physiological functioning.

The Tyranny of Bad Habits

The enervated and toxemic from established bad habits thinks, because he once ate to excess, ate wrong combinations, and used stimulants of all kinds, that he can continue to do so, and a curing system that cannot restore him to health, and leave him alone to enjoy his disease-building habits, is certainly no good and should be branded Kill-Joy. The very scientific bacteriological plan of vaccination and serum inoculation is supposed to cure and immunize the dear people, and leave them alone to enjoy life to its fullest extent, without any danger of coming down with disease. The *reliability* of this system, carried out under compulsion, has been observed in the various cantonments during the fall and winter of 1917 and 1918; also the standard of health of America may be offered as "Exhibit I" in testimony of the virtue of a system that cures without removing cause.

Enzymes (Digestive Ferments)

The stomach and bowels liquify the foods taken into them by virtue of the enzymes (unorganized ferments) secreted into them by secretory glands. Every organ and tissue in the body has an enzyme all its own, which is necessary to prepare the building material selected from the circulating fluid.

[85]

When there is a shortage of these enzymes, the renewal of tissue will be imperfect. For example: When the blood, which is a fluid organ, is waterlogged, its enzymic supply is weakened by bacterial infection coming from the fermentation in the bowels. The result of this infection is that the blood is unable to select the mineral elements necessary for corpuscle-building. Without iron, blood corpuscles cannot be built. When iron cannot be appropriated and red corpuscles built, there must be oxygen starvation; and when the other minerals cannot be appropriated, various other starvations take place. Starvation is not so much a question of lack of food as of a lack of power to appropriate it. Abuse of eating and drinking, and lack of mental poise, start the gastric fermentation which is the cause of all causes of perverted health.

We should remember that there is no disease *per se*—only impaired health.

Exercise Is Necessary

The intake of food must be balanced by a proper amount of exercise; but when an excess of either or both has been indulged in for a few years, great care, and even skill, is sometimes required in readjusting, or harm will follow. Those who have lived sedentary lives, neglecting exercise, fresh air, and sunshine, will suffer greatly if suddenly changed from sedentary indoor life to an active outdoor life, and *vice versa.*

OVERDEVELOPMENT

Athletes seldom die of old age. Brawn does not necessarily mean health. All who boast of hard muscles, and are considered in the prime of health, even by most doctors — yes even by doctors who pretend to judge of the physical status of athletes—are toxin-poisoned from overeating and wrong food combinations. With them disease is imminent, and will take hold of them as soon as they retire from active training. Those with diathesis (predispositions to develop certain diseases) will develop tuberculosis, Bright's disease, arterial, heart, or circuatory diseases, such as hardening of the arteries, endocarditis, apoplexy, paralysis, etc.; others will develop gouty diseases, such as rheumatism, stone in the gall-bladder, in the kidney, urinary bladder, etc. This is why the athlete never "comes back." The man of the gouty diathesis is stiffened with disease, so that he has lost all of his resiliency; like Lot's wife, he is turned into a pillar of salt—a punishment for looking back on a passive life, and continuing the sensuality practiced during the active life. Even in the commonplace affairs of life we see those who give up an active for a passive life going down and out. When the farmer retires, his retirement is often the beginning of the end of h e a l t h . Nature abhors sudden changes, and the greater the physical development, the greater the reaction when training ceases.

Moderation is written all over the face of nature, and the eternal fiat has gone out that he who deviates from the order punishes himself in keeping with his deviation.

All the old men and women with whom I have had the pleasure of an acquaintance have told me that, while they have not abstained from convention's sensuality, they have indulged very moderately. One man, who has always commanded my respect for his all-round good sense, confessed to me at one time, with a twinkle in his more than seventy-year-old eyes: "Doctor, I have always indulged myself moderately in all the petty vices common to gentlemen."

What Is Moderation?

Moderation is indulgence that does not overtax and interfere with metabolism (tissue change). Overstimulation from food, drinks, work, play, and joy, when continued, enervates. And an enervated body cannot take care of itself—it fails to clean house, and the standard of health is lowered. This is called disease.

What is moderation for one is overindulgence for another. No one can gauge his limitations by the limitation of others. What someone else eats, and apparently gets away with, is no gauge for anybody else. Every being is a law unto himself. When it comes to eating and indulging sense, it is not what convention says; it is not what the family physician or the specialist says; it is what the being's sensations tell him. Discomfort of the slightest nature following indulgence should receive attention, and moderation or abstinence will be adopted by the prudent. Those who are not prudent will rush on to discomfort, pain, and death.

To live in such a way as to be comfortable all the time; free from the little sicknesses *common to good society;* free from overweight or underweight; free from bad odors from breath or body; free from the ugliness of skin that requires constant veneering to keep it from the public gaze; to have a mind that is alert and progressive, not afraid of new thought, and that can see the absurdity of clinging to the old simply because of respectability, or because the majority do it; to be afraid of ignorance—this is living moderately and wholesomely.

Living penuriously, as well as living extravagantly, is unwise. Fanaticism turns loose in the blood toxins that dwarf the mind and harden the arteries. The same may be said of overworking the emotions.

Today wise men are honest; for it is the most economical thing to do.

John Barleycorn has been knocked out by his former friends. Enough people have learned that, if they would get on in the world, they must part company with alcoholics, to cause the whole country to "go dry." There are many still standing in their own light by bootlegging—adding crime to drinking. Both must lead to waste of energy, premature aging, and early death, besides handicapping efficiency and sidestepping self-respect and success.

Overstimulation

Alcohol, tobacco, coffee, tea, overeating, extravagant ideas and overuse of the imagination and the nerves of special sense, lead to enervation, impaired health, and early death.

There is no moderate ground for stimulation. One person may be more moderate than another; yet the one who indulges a little in any of the conventional vices will curtail his life. He may live to be called "a grand old man"* yet he dies years too soon and weakens his efficiency to the extent that men with half his experience take his place in the world's work. Why? Is it because age impairs judgment? No; age does not impair judgment, but stimulants do. Drivel and senility is not old age; for it is seen in middle age and sometimes youth. It is disease and bad habits.

*The popular estimate is capricious, and always questionable and low.

Alcohol hardens tissue. It hardens the liver. If it hardens the liver, it must harden the brain—the cerebro-spinal centers are hardened, and necessarily the brain and cord functions are impaired. A little impairment handicaps judgment, and is liable to write failure across man's life, when it would have been a success without the stimulant.

Overstimulation in the first half of life may show, as sequels, imbecility, epilepsy, infantile paralysis, or other nervous diseases in the children. These sequels may appear in children twenty years after reform has taken place in the parents.

A respectable banker, preacher, doctor, or lawyer, advanced to young-old age, may be forced to see the sequel of his early indiscretions developing before him in the shape of children with such profound nervous diatheses that they have little resistance to disease-producing influences. When transmitted diatheses—tendencies to take on disease—are understood, then we have the reason why so many children come down with infantile paralysis after a prolonged season of enervating weather. Certain atmospheric states of a stimulating or depressing character do come about almost, if not quite, every year—states of prolonged dry, wet, hot, cold, or windy weather. It is then that diathetic subjects, weighed down to the breaking point with unfavorable personal and domestic influences and habits, require only "the last straw" to cause them to give down and develop a disease in keeping with the influence complex— the sum of the compound influences. Where the influences are spent on a neurotic child, infantile paralysis or some other nervous disease develops; where the subject is of the tuberculosis diathesis, tuberculosis will develop; etc.

People of vital temperament have more resistance and can stand more stimulation. Those who advocate the idea that a specific germ is the cause of all diseases will hoot at my explanation of the cause of disease. We must not forget, however, that owls hoot in the dark; when brought into the light they stop their hooting. Suffice it to say that no children develop convulsions, paralysis, or nervous diseases who do not inherit tendencies which can be traced to parents or grandparents. The same is true of all other diatheses.

Moderation of Inheritance

Certainly no one who thinks would expect a child with a nervous diathesis to thrive on excitement and stimulants. Indeed, such children must be carefully managed and screened from overstimulation. They must not be overfed; their food should be the most simple; and their play must be devoid of the nerve-wrecking noise and activity often indulged in by strong, healthy children.

Prospective parents must invoice their stock of health. If they find that in their parents or grandparents there are qualities of mind or body which are not desirable to have transmitted to their children, it is their duty to do all they can to build themselves up. Then, when the children come, everything must be done to encourage body-building; for certainly everything that tends to lower the vitality of the child favors the development of the diseases peculiar to the inherited tendencies.

Much can be done to suppress inherited tendencies. A child marked with inebriating tendencies certainly should be kept from stimulants. It should be understood that excess in any way means overstimulation. For example, the child of a drunken father should be kept away from alcoholics, and it should be guarded against every other excess; for excesses of all kinds lead to the Rome of intemperance. While some excesses are worse than others, yet it is desirable to avoid intemperance of all kinds. The drunkard's child may be so prejudiced against drink that its prejudice becomes a ruinous fanaticism. The child of a debauchee* is inclined to develop debauchery of mind or body—go to excess, to extremes, in sensual pleasures—and become handicapped for life by them. This tendency, where it exists, must be held before the child's mind, and the fatality of the tendency, if indulged, must be explained. Great moderation is the only safe plan after the dangers of heredity are understood.

The false belief is quite general, that, if children are kept from alcoholics, tobacco, onanism, etc., when matured into manhood and womanhood they will be safe—no danger of their taking

*From a medical standpoint, debauchery should mean excess in any line of stimulation. There are more food drunkards than any other class, except venereal.

on these habits. The Bible students believe that "the way the twig is bent the tree inclines," and if the child is "brought up in the fear and admonition of the Lord," it will not depart from the teachings when it is old. I have observed people taking up the tobacco and alcohol habits after middle life. One man with whom I was acquainted did not know the taste of whisky at forty years of age, yet he died from drunkenness in less than fifteen years after he started the habit. It is common to see men using tobacco for the first time after forty to fifty years of age. They are all inebriates of some kind—most of them food drunkards.

The question, after all, is that of understanding. Moderation in a few things and intemperance in others is not a reliable way to build character. The preacher may admonish his family regarding the evils of the customs of the *fast set*, and at the same time cultivate a morbid intolerance for those who hold opinions contrary to his; in other words, cultivate a bigotry and fanaticism that kills sweet love and charity, and at the same time cultivate such food drunkenness that he dies in middle life from lung, kidney, or heart disease, or from ulcer or cancer of the stomach or bowels. And, because of his licentious indulgence in allowable habits, he transmits to posterity a diathesis that favors the development of disease and crime.

A gluttonous father is represented by a drunken son, a sordid wealth-gatherer may be followed by a son with criminal tendencies; a sensual father often begets a tuberculous son —bacteriology to the contrary.

The greatest legacy that can be left to children is a sound constitution. Certainly no one is so short of good sense and logic as to believe that those who overindulge in any sensual way can impart ideal constitutions to their children.

If the race is to be improved, it cannot be done so long as tuberculosis, *is caused by germs*, and the habits of children and parents are of no importance.

Few know all they should about their inherited tendencies. The tendency of many people to pedestalize their relatives inclines them to be conceited about their inheritances. Because of this conceit, they are often destined to a very rude awakening, when a son turns out a drunkard or an absconder, or a beautiful daughter develops into a cleptomanic or ducks out of sight with some good-for-nothing. These phenomena are not accidents; they are as exact as the workingout of geometrical problems—they are the resultant of excess in parents and grandparents, and overindulgence of the children. Excessive indulgence of children fills the hospitals, insane asylums, reform schools, jails, and penitentiaries.

Prospective parents should not indulge the notion that the practice of excess in secret will not be declared on the housetops by either themselves or their children.

The beginning of sensuality is at the mother's breast. The first gastritis, cold, or cholera infantum—the first sick spell that baby has after birth —is the sequel of baby's first debauch. Every sick spell thereafter is a crisis developing in the course of a chronic blood derangement fed by fermentation. Infantile acidosis, continued, becomes toxemia in adults, and all the common diseases are crises—legitimate developments in the course of a life of overindulgence and chronic toxemia. Food drunkenness is as fixed a type of debauchery as alcohol drunkenness or any other form of health-destroying habits.

So little is generally known of the influence of food on health that it may be recognized as the decoy that leads to ruin. Food is necessary to our existence; and shallow minds declare, not only that it is necessary, but the more the better—that it is necessary to eat heartily (which means excessively) to keep up the strength.

When food excess has been indulged in for years, it fails to satisfy. This overstimulation, like all other excesses, calls for other stimulation. It is then easy to develop the tobacco, alcohol, and other drug habits; for one form of excess leads to other forms.

Excessive eating leads on and on to sickness, sorrow, pain, and death.

Haphazard Eating

Next to overeating as a cause of disease is the indiscriminate eating seen everywhere. People are advertised as "good livers" who exhibit a wild haphazard in setting their tables. Hotels and eating-houses secure the enviable reputation of "setting good tables'' if they overload them with bread and a half-dozen other pronounced starches, such as potatoes, rice, navy or butter beans, spaghetti, tapioca, bread pudding, *et al*. It is common to see six decidedly starchy foods on a *well supplied* table, and often several kinds of meat.

All the authority which people have for eating haphazardly — for eating from ten to twenty varieties of food at a meal—is that the best and most informed do so; everybody who can afford it does so; and those who cannot afford it go as far as they can in imitation of the plan.

CONSEQUENCE

Disease is as common as abominable eating. To be sick; to be ailing; to be complaining; to have headaches, neuralgia, rheumatic pains; large, sensitive, and deformed knuckles; impaired eyesight; thick, muddy skin; ugly complexion, a breath that is disagreeable; a temper and disposition that make life a weary dream—these are a few of the many discomforts which people ignorantly saddle upon themselves because of blindly following in the wake of custom in eating; going on the principle that ''what was good enough for my father and mother is good enough for me." Indeed, every generation should demand better developing knowledge. We should strive for efficiency. Simply to exist is not all that man should want. Animals can live that life; but man should be unfolding.

Germs a Cause of Disease

The masses excuse themselves for being sick; for it is the popular opinion that invisible germs cause disease, and, of course, it is impossible for laymen to avoid their sickness-producing influence.

This is a false understanding of the influence of germs on human health and life. Germs can have no sickness-producing influence on those who are well—in full health. What is meant by "full health"? Full resistance to germ influence does not necessarily mean a well-trained brawn. To be a gladiator does not mean power to resist germs. Few physical experts—athletes—live to be old, because they eat in a manner to keep themselves toxin-poisoned; and this, too, in spite of their great muscle development and strength of body.

The hibernating animal gets rid of germs and toxins while hibernating; the sick get rid of germs when fasting for a sufficient length of time. This being true, then germs are not *per se* the cause of disease. If they were man's enemy, they would take advantage of his weakened and starved state to do their worst; but they thrive best in the strong, overfed, and overindulged.

Thousands of our soldier boys could boast of never having been ill before they were vaccinated, inoculated, serumated, overclothed, and fed on meat, potatoes, bread, and coffee three times a day; after which they were knocked down with pneumonia, measles, scarlet fever, meningitis, typhoid fever, etc.

Disease comes from an oversupply of food, which must break down, rot, and pass out of the body. While this is going on, toxins are formed, absorbed, and for a time cause sickness. But if no more food be taken, then putrefaction comes to an end with the toxin infection and germ multiplication.

If germs were the cause of disease, only the weak and fasting would be subject to their influence. But exactly the reverse is true. Only the overfed, be they strong or weak, are carriers of germs; and they become victims of disease when vaccinated, inoculated, or otherwise immunized, because every such act lowers resistance. Then, if they are huddled together as men and women are in our theatres, lecture-halls, and places of amusement, so-called contagious diseases take hold of all who are below a certain stand-ard of resistance. Or perhaps it would be nearer the truth to say that all will be prostrated with disease who have organic diatheses. The organ affected individualizes the type of disease. Where there is a tendency for skin disease, the sum of the influences will evolve an exanthema; where the lungs are the vulnerable organs, a pneu-monia evolves; where the cerebro-spinal system is most vulnerable, in-fantile paralysis, meningitis, etc., will develop.

Athletes Die Early

Why do pugilists die early—why do athletes generally die early? Because they have the overeating habit; and intestinal putrefaction always accompanies overeating. This means that their bodies are repositories for an excess of bacteria—germs of fermentation. As soon as they stop forcing, by heavy exercise, an intake of a surplus of oxygen with which to oxidize and neutralize the excess of carbon-dioxide and other products of metabolism, they develop a sick habit and begin their march toward physical disintegration.

Obesity

Obesity is the result of wrong eating. The excessive intake of carbohydrate foods—starch and sugar—and fat, builds obesity. Where the excess weight is not an inheritance, it should be looked upon as disease, and should be treated as such; but where the stoutness is a diethesis—where the tendency to grow "too stout" is inherited—it is not to be got rid of, but should be controlled. The diathetically obese—those born to be fat—must be educated into aknowledge of how to live to prevent burdening their vital organs with an accumulation of fat. These subjects should be round and sleek, but not burdened. Double chins and rolls of fat on the back of the neck and head are danger signs and should be heeded. Men of this type may weigh two and a half pounds to the inch of stature without jeopardizing health and life, and women may weigh from two to two and a quarter pounds to the inch — an amount of weight that would be dangerous to those who have not an inherited tendency to be stout.

Those who develop excess weight without an inherited diathesis must take advice and be on the alert to ward off kidney or heart affections, and certainly must eschew stimulants of all kinds.

To control weight, starch must be given up entirely for a time; then it may be used in great moderation for one meal a day. It should be taken in the form of thoroughly toasted bread; or, occasionally, well cooked oatmeal or other breakfast foods. The obese should live largely on succulent vegetables and fresh, uncooked fruits.

The Excessively Lean

To be underweight is a sign of perverted health. Women may weigh one and a half pounds to the inch of stature and not be underweight. Men are usually underweight if they weigh less than two pounds to the inch. This is true of tall men, but not of short men. A six-foot man is getting rather thin when weighing below one hundred and forty-five pounds; yet there are men enjoying excellent health who weigh less than two pounds to the inch.

Weight should not receive much attention. The requirement for health should be a bright eye, an active mind, a clear skin, and a willowy body. These all indicate the best of health, even if the weight should be less than one and a half pounds to the inch.

The average layman is ignorant enough to thing that unless a human being is fat unto death—in the condition of stock-show animals—he is not in prime condition.

Weight that prevents activity, causes sleepiness, and is accompanied with bad breath and discomforts of any kind, should be reduced.

Eating correctly in the line of proper combinations, and avoiding overeating, with proper bathing, clothing, and exercise, plus a poised mind, will build ideal health; and the weight will be neither over nor under the proper standard for the individual.

Self-Protection

The best self-protection is to understand how to eat so as to avoid the fermentation and decomposition which follow improper food combinations and overeating. This little Dietitian can help anyone to a safe knowledge of *how to eat for health.*

———◆———

No science is so full of fallacies, errors, illusions, and lies as the school of medicine.—Dr. Richter, M.D.

• • •

No systematic or theoretical classification of diseases or therapeutical agents ever yet promulgated is true.—Sir John Forbes, F.R.C.P., London.

• • •

Medicine is cranky and irrational, more dangerous than dynamite.— J. N. Hurty, M.D., Indiana State Board of Health.

• • •

There is not a single medicine in all the world which does not carry harm in its molecules.—J. H. Hurty, M.D., Indiana State Board of Heath.

[107]

An Object Lesson

A FEW DINNER MENUS FROM THE DINING
ROOM OF THE TILDEN HEALTH SCHOOL

1
Lima beans
Stewed celery, cabbage
Grapefruit

2
Tomato soup
Veal
Turnips, string beans
Salad
Fruit Jello

3
Baked squash
Peas and string beans
Parsnips
Salad

4
Celery soup
Baked Irish potatoes
Onions, carrots
Salad

5
Vegetable soup
Pecans (30 half nut meats), Raisins
Cottage cheese
Stewed tomatoes, cabbage
Salad

6

Baked sweet potatoes
Peas, turnips
Salad

7

Tomato soup
Baked halibut
Peach and apple sauce
Carrots, stewed tomatoes
Grapefruit

8

Celery soup
Baked sweet potatoes
Corn, cabbage
Salad

9

Christmas Dinner

Tomato soup
Celery, olives
Roast turkey, giblet gravy
Cranberry sauce
Jelly
Turnips and carrots
String beans
Salad
Mince pie
Nuts, raisins, figs

10

Tomato soup
Belgian hare
Turnips and parsnips
Peas
Currant jelly
Caramel custard

11

Celery soup
Corn bread
Parsnips, beets
Salad

12

Hominy
Beets, onions
Salad

13

Roast beef
Peas and carrots
Stewed tomatoes
Grapefruit

14

Baked squash
Parsnips, corn
Salad

15

Steamed eggs, bacon
String beans
Turnips
Grapefruit

CPSIA information can be obtained
at www.ICGtesting.com
Printed in the USA
LVOW03s1443150516

488340LV00022BA/655/P